Migraine Relief

Eliminate Migraine Pain Using Essential Oils and Aromatherapy

Emily V. Steinhauser

Want a Free E-Book?

Signup for the Gamma Mouse Media Newsletter and pick a free e-book as a Thank You Gift.

For more details and to sign-up, visit http://www.gammamouse.com.

What You Need to Know about Migraine Headaches

Understanding migraines and its headaches are the second most sought for services after tension headaches. Migraines headaches run in families as a result of heredity. The Migraines disease attacks are more common in individuals between the age of 20 - 30 years. However, the age at which one may start feeling these headaches may vary though it is very rare in older ages.

Types of Migraines

1. Common migraines. These are migraines without Aura

2. Migraines with Aura

3. Hemiplegic migraines

4. Basilar artery migraines

5. Retinal migraines

6. Ophthalmologic migraines

7. Abdominal migraines

Symptoms of Migraines

Migraines attack symptoms differ from one individual to another. Migraines has four phases of attack, however, not all of these phases occur in migraines victims.

1. Prodrome Migraines Phase

The prodrome signs and symptoms occur in approximately 40-60% of all migraines victims. The symptoms in this phase include irritability, altered mood, yawning, fatigue and craving for certain types of food. These symptoms normally precede several hours of headaches.

2. The Aura Migraines Phase

In this stage, migraines victims experiences auras that are either in form of sensory, visual or motor disturbances. Visual auras are however more common in this phase. Visual destructions include zigzag lines, flashes of light and cloud vision. However, these auras do not last for more than an hour.

3. Headache Phase

Migraines headaches can be extremely severe lasting for more than 3 hours and go as long as three days. These headaches are normally accompanied by nausea and vomiting. Migraines sufferers in this stage will only get peace and comfort if they only sleep in a quiet and dark room.

4. Postdrome Phase

This is the last phase of migraines where patients normally feel weak and tired. This phase is also called the "hangover" phase.

There are so many factors that can lead one to have a migraines attack. The most common causes of migraines attack include:

a) Changes in sleep pattern

b) Physical, mental or emotional stress

c) Weather changes

d) Loud noises, bright lights to certain odour

e) Exposure to smoke or smoking

f) Alcohol

g) Certain foods such as aged cheese, red wine, monosodium glutamate, chocolates, banana, citrus, onions , dairy products and nitrates in salami, bacon and sausages.

Migraines Management

Migraines management involves avoiding future triggers and taking prophylactic medication to prevent future attacks. Management of migraines is majorly centered on treating the migraines headaches.

How to Treat Acute Migraines

i. Use Ergot derivatives. Ergot derivatives such as Ergotamine are used as rescue medication for acute migraines attacks.

ii. You can also take pain killers. A good example here is the paracetamol drug which you can use with or without relaxant. You can also use anti-inflammatory and non- steroidal drugs to relief pain, and add an anti-vomiting drug to stop nausea.

iii. Triptans such as naratriptan, sumatriptan, eletriptan and zolmitriptan can also help you to abort acute migraines attacks.

Prophylactic treatment

Prophylactic treatment is a preventive form of treatment. You should always consult your doctor before starting prophylactic treatment mostly if you are having frequent headaches. Prophylaxis treatment can use a wide range of medicine such as calcium channel blockers, beta blockers, antidepressants, NSAIDS, anticonvulsants and angiotensins.

All in all, understanding migraines require a "migraines diary". This diary will help you in identifying possible migraines triggers. Without knowing these triggers it will be extremely difficult to avoid them.

The Various Causes of Migraines

Migraine is a disorder affect the nervous system. It is characterized by moderate to severe headaches that normally affect one side of the head. The headaches are osscilative in nature and may last from 2 to 72 hours. Other symptoms of migraines may include: nausea, fatigue, numbness, vomiting and sensitivity to sound, light and smell.

They are believed to be due to a mixture of environmental and genetic factors. The exact causes of migraines are unknown but professional medics have narrowed down to some of the things that are believed to trigger migraines. Below are some of the common triggers of migraines.

Diet.

Some foods can trigger migraines examples of these are; aged cheeses, chocolate, nuts, citrus fruits, soy foods, vinegar etc. Poor nutrition, magnesium deficiency, lack of B vitamins and irregular feeding patterns are also migraine triggers.

It is therefore advisable to avoid or minimize intake of such foods to avoid migraines. It is also important to have a regular feeding strategy and take a well-balanced diet.

Alcohol.

Beer, red wine, etc contain tyramine in large amounts. Tiggeryramine is one of the most powerful migraine triggers. Alcohol also causes dehydration which is also a migraine trigger.

Extreme temperature changes.

You may be inside a conditioned room during a hot day and when you get out you may experience sudden extreme temperature changes. Or taking a hot shower then moving into cold weather. These sudden temperature changes can trigger migraines.

High sensory stimuli.

Bright light, loud noises and strong smells can trigger migraines. It is therefore advisable to avoid intense stimuli.

Stress.

When one is stressed the body reacts physically with hormonal elevation and tension of muscles. These changes can trigger migraines. It is therefore advisable to avoid stress as much as possible.

Medications.

Some medications such as antihistamines, oral contraceptives, decongestants, blood pressure medications and hormone replacement drugs may trigger migraines.

Hormonal changes.

Estrogen and progesterone hormones are potential causes of migraines. This is the reason why women are at a higher risk of having migraines. Hormonal changes during menstruation, pregnancy or menopause may trigger migraines.

Changes in sleeping patterns.

Sleep is the best form of resting and all humans need to relax and have a good sleep every day. Lack of enough sleep or irregular sleeping patterns causes straining of brain cell which can easily trigger migraines.

Too much sleep is also a trigger of migraines. It is therefore advisable to have just enough sleep every day to avoid migraines.

Genes.

Researchers suspect that migraines may be triggered by an inherited gene therefore having a family member who has migraines may increase your chances of having migraines.

Physical straining.

Extreme physical activities, muscle straining and even sexual activity may trigger migraines. Avoid too much physical activity and always take a rest whenever you feel that you need to.

Dehydration

The human body requires to maintain certain amounts of fluid within the tissues. If the level of body fluid is lower than the required, one is said to be dehydrated and is at a high risk of migraine.

It is advisable to take enough water and to avoid alcohol which may lead to dehydration.

Poor posture.

Postures that cause tension of the neck and shoulders may also trigger migraines. Always ensure that you assume postures that feel comfortable.

These are some are some of the most common causes of migraines and where possible, one should avoid these triggers for a healthy life.

Basic Medical Treatments for Migraines

There's no denying it - migraines are horrible. Anyone who has ever had them can tell you how debilitating they can be. Some lucky people, among those who are unlucky enough to get migraines in the first place, only get them infrequently, maybe a couple of times a month, while other are inundated with them day after day. Whatever your particular circumstances are, if you get migraines, you can be sure that you want to get rid of them, and are a few tips regarding the best treatment of migraines.

1. Take OTC Medications Containing Aspirin and Codeine

Aspirin is generally considered to be more effective for migraines than other, similar medications such as acetaminophen (Tylenol) and ibuprofen (Advil). Some preparations combine Aspirin with codeine, which can make it even more effective still. Aspirin works to thin the blood and reduce blood pressure, while the opiate codeine works synergistically to reduce pain further.

The only problem with this sort of treatment is that it treats the symptoms instead of the cause. If your migraines are frequent, then your body may adjust to the codeine and it may no longer be efficacious, as well as causing a rebound headache. These kind of medications tend to be most effective if you take it just when a migraine starts.

2. See Your Doctor about Preventative Medications

If you find yourself turning to OTC drugs too often, especially in cases of frequent/daily migraines, you might want to book an appointment with your doctor to get something that prevents them from happening altogether. There are a variety of medications available, and your doctor will be able to steer you towards the right one.

3. Get a Massage, Especially For the Neck

People who get migraines will notice a stiffness and soreness around the neck. Some of this muscular tension and stress can be relieved by getting a vigorous massage. Though it may seem like a luxury to some, such massages are highly beneficial for migraine headaches, and often come recommended from doctors.

4. Put a Hot Towel around Your Neck

Similar to a massage, a towel soaked with hot water rested on the neck can help relieve muscle tension, as well as reducing the pain of the migraine itself.

5. If Possible, Lie in a Dark, Quiet Room

If you're at work, this isn't likely to be an option, but if you're at home when a headache strikes, many people intuitively find that moving away from light and noise helps. A bedroom with the blinds drawn and the lights off is the perfect place, because, if you're lucky, you may be able to sleep it out, and wake with the migraine having passed.

Many people will likely have various bits of advice about the treatment of migraines, advising you to avoid certain triggers such as stress, sugar, and so on. You may want to look further into this, and discuss with your doctor what triggers may be the cause and how to best go about avoiding them. In the meantime, though, the strategies above for the treatment of migraines should provide some much needed relief.

Using Aromatherapy to Treat Migraines

People who suffer from migraines are often subjected to debilitating pain that makes it difficult to complete many ordinary activities. Going to work, attending school or taking care of normal household responsibilities can prove next to impossible.

Unfortunately, many conventional doctors prescribe pain medications that only dull the pain that migraines cause, while failing to address the sense of anxiety and other symptoms that people experience as their headaches are building.

These medications are rarely capable of limiting the frequency of migraines and in some instances, they may not lessen the severity. More importantly, most pharmaceutical products entail a range of side effects that are just as unpleasant as the problems they are meant to treat. This is why many people are currently using aromatherapy to treat migraines in conjunction with other nature-based remedies.

Different Ways in Which Using Aromatherapy to Treat Migraines Can Provide Relief

There are many ways in which using aromatherapy to treat migraines can lessen the panic and discomfort that are associated with this issue. It is important to note that most people view aromatherapy as a good supplementary treatment for migraines rather than as a primary or sole solution.

Using essential oils for physiological and psychological relief is something that people can do on their own or under the guidance of a naturopath or other alternative medicine specialists. These remedies can be used in conjunction with chiropractic care, acupuncture or even more conventional treatments.

The most common way to use aromatherapy for migraines is with the goal of creating a calming effect. Increased anxiety during the building stage of a migraine can intensify the headache and extend its duration.

Secondary symptoms such as nausea, sleeplessness, congestion and depression can be alleviated through the use of aromatic essential oils as well. Red mandarin and lemongrass oils are great for alleviating depression. Peppermint oil can stave off migraine-related nausea and clary sage oils can relieve an increasing sense of panic. Facial pain and sinus congestion often respond positively to eucalyptus oils.

Important Things to Remember When Using Essential Oils to Treat Migraines

It is vital for people to know that some essential oils can actually act as triggers for migraines. Thus, those who are new to aromatherapy may want to seek professional guidance in choosing the right essential oils, carrier oils and oil blends for achieving desirable results.

People must also be cognizant of the fact that this type of therapy is most effective when implemented during the migraine building stage and as part of an integrated plan for making the migraine abate.

Using Carrier Oils

In spite of their pleasing fragrances, the potency of essential oils should never be underestimated. These oils have the potential to burn soft tissues and cause irritation to the eyes and airways, especially when there is direct and prolonged exposure. For this reason, all essential oils must first be tempered with an acceptable carrier oil such as coconut oil, grapeseed or almond oil.

They must also be disbursed in the appropriate fashion, whether through aroma diffusers and lamps, smelling salts or pre-bottled blends. With the right tempering strategies and selection of oils, using aromatherapy to treat migraines is a great way to quickly gain an increased sense of relief without experiencing negative and unpleasant side effects.

Treating Migraines Using Essential Oils

Essential oils are special oils that are extracted from plant natural sources. They contain volatile aromatic compounds that give them their characteristic fragrant smell(s) which depends on the plant source that they were extracted from. Apart from their attractive smells, essential oils have found many medical uses and are a rich source of therapeutics that is yet to be fully exploited.

The most outstanding use of essential oils is their application in the management of migraines; neurological disorder that is characterized by repeated episodes of mild to severe headaches and other symptoms of disorder of the autonomic nervous system.

Mechanism of action of essential oils

The broad spectrum of use of essential oil in the medical field is based on their diverse mechanism(s) of action. Critical to the management of migraines is their potency to relieve anxiety, stabilize moods and process of moods change, sedate the brain hence induce some sleep, lower blood pressure and pain.

These are the main benefits of essential oils when it comes to the management of migraines but it doesn't stop at this. Some can also be used as accelerators of wound healing process, antiseptics, perfumery and food spices.

Key examples of essential oils that are used for management of migraine are;

Eucalyptus oil: This is the most widely used essential oil in the management of migraines. The oil is extracted from the fresh leaves of eucalyptus trees but mainly from Eucalyptus globulus. The oil is transparent or might have a little brown tint depending on the degree of purity. Its fragrance is irresistible and this arises from the cooling and refreshing effect that it gives upon inhalation of its aroma.

The oil is actually a mental stimulant that alleviates all your mental pressure, stress and fatigue which more than often are contributors to migraine.

The oil can be administered by rubbing on the scalp and the whole head or inhaling fumes of the oil for a few minutes. This can be done at intervals until the migraine relieving effects of the oil are achieved.

Lavender essential oil: This oil is common in many places and is extracted from the flower spikes of lavender. Just like many other essential oils it's colorless.

For production of migraine relieving effects, the oil is administered the same way as eucalyptus oil above. This oil is most suitable for use during the night hours.

Peppermint essential oil: This oil contains menthol as the main ingredient. Menthol has been known for many years for its mind relaxing effects.

It gives a general good feeling of eased muscular tension and fatigue as well as pain alleviation. The oil is a central nervous system stimulant and may interfere with sleep.

Chamomile essential oil: Many varieties of this oil exist but the only ones used with migraines are- Roman and the German. This oil is extracted from the flower-heads of Chamaemelum nobile. The oil is common in many parts of the world and its use in the management of migraines cannot be nullified.

Other major essential oils used in the management of migraines are; Cinnamon oil, Basil oil, Carrot seed oil, Pine oil and Citronella oil.

Safety of essential oil in migraine management

Essential oils are very safe for use because they have minimal side effects if any. They are inert to the skin and do not cause any irritation or adverse reactions. Most of them are inhaled as fumes without causing any respiratory irritation or side effects. Important to note is their intrinsic capability to interfere with sleeping because some of them are central nervous system stimulants such as the eucalyptus oil.

The migraine relieving effects of essential oils are incomparable to any other migraine therapy in the market today and they should give you a permanent solution to your migraine problem. Try them today and your migraine will go away forever.

Thank You!

I hope you have found this guide to migraine relief to be helpful and informative. Migraines are a terrible thing to have to deal with so if this guide is able to help ease your pain, it is terribly worth it to me. I wish you all the success in dispelling these debilitating headaches.

Good luck!

Free Bonus Book

Thank you so much for your purchase. As an additional bonus we are including another great book, Ketogenic Diet by Nicole Harrington for you.

I hope you enjoy!

Ketogenic Diet

The Effective and Safe Way to Lose
Weight and Regain Your Life

Nicole Harrington

First Edition: June 2014
123456789
Published by Gamma Mouse
http://gammamouse.com

This document is geared towards providing exact and reliable information in regards to the topic and issue covered. The publication is sold with the idea that the publisher is not required to render accounting, officially permitted, or otherwise, qualified services. If advice is necessary, legal or professional, a practiced individual in the profession should be ordered.

From a Declaration of Principles which was accepted and approved equally by a Committee of the American Bar Association and a Committee of Publishers and Associations.

The information provided herein is stated to be truthful and consistent, in that any liability, in terms of inattention or otherwise, by any usage or abuse of any

The Amazing Ketogenic Diet

The idea of ketogenic dieting is not peculiar. As a matter of facts, ketogenic diet has been there in many forms and in many variations. It has got many similarities to the Atkins diet. By the end of this article, you will be able to find what exactly ketogenic diet is, how and reasons why it works. Otherwise, it is good to note that, ketogenic exists in three different types: the Targeted ketogenic diet, cyclical ketogenic diet and the Standard Ketogenic diet. They are almost the same but differ according to limits and timing of carbohydrates consumption.

So, what is the Ketogenic diet?

In simple terms, ketogenic diet can be defined as any diet that forces the body in a process known as the Ketosis, whereby extra fats are burned as an alternative of carbohydrates which is used as energy. The right ketogenic diet requires the dieter to consume high amount of fat, sufficient amounts of protein and very small amounts of carbohydrates. It is also good to note that, bodies are of the character that, they turn extra carbohydrate in glucose which is sent to all over the body in energy form. When you enter ketosis by sufficiently restricting your carbohydrate consumption, your livers begin breaking down fat cells into fatty acids and ketones, which is supposed to be used as the energy.

How does ketogenic diet work?

Just like any other diet that you know of, ketogenic diet works by reducing the amount of calories you consume, in turn creates a caloric shortfall where the body burns more energy than it takes. That is the basic science of weight loss, and even though the argument is subjected to further debating, few shall be of the opinion that, all successful diets depends on caloric limitation, in one way or another. The following are some of the advantages of ketogenic diet:

It helps in controlling blood sugar and minimizing insulin spikes

When you consume carbohydrates, your blood sugar level would increase tremendously; this will also cause the fast insulin reaction from the pancreatic gland. This insulin is useful in dispersing excess blood glucose, which makes you to feel hungry almost immediately. And if you eat a low carbohydrate diet, you succeed in keeping your blood sugar levels low and hence the carb that induces hunger spikes are avoided. Reducing hormone level is the top priority for any diet so does ketogenic diet. Insulin should be reduced because it is the hormone that induces the body to store fat.

Ketogenic diet enables the body consume food that is satiating and filling

Those who have eaten ketogenic diet do find it extremely easy to limit calories. If you are using this diet in the right way, you will be able to consume quite a good amount of calories daily ranging from fats to protein which is both satiating and scrumptious. Those are in ketogenic diet would find it hard to consume enough food every day.

Finally, ketogenic diets have become more popular for many reasons. A part from helping weight loss, it is being considered as the possible treatment or prevention of epilepsy and researches have also shown that it can also be used in neurological conditions. Having known what the ketogenic diet is, you can try it if you have used it and you will be dumbfounded. Ketogenic diet is highly recommended.

Is the Ketogenic Diet Right For Me?

Benefits of the Ketogenic Diet

The benefits if ketogenic diet are numerous and happy ones. Some of the benefits one may expect after switching to ketogenic diet include:

It is always important to get a full blood lipid panel before starting on this diet so one can compare their blood work after starting on the diet.

Lower blood pressure

Ketogenic diets are effective in lowering the blood pressure. Though, if one is taking blood pressure medication, they should be aware that they begin to feel dizzy or tipsy from too much medication while on this diet. It is advisable for people suffering from blood pressure related diseases to seek a doctor's advice before starting on this diet

A drop in cholesterol

Cholesterol is usually made out of excess glucose. This diet requires one to consume less sugar foods which simply mean a reduction in the excess glucose. The body cholesterol will drop as the body has less glucose to make cholesterol

A drop in triglycerides

Consumption of carbohydrates is closely attached to triglycerides levels. This is the most well-known ketogenic diet advantage. The less the carbohydrates consumed, the lower the triglycerides readings will go. The triglycerides: HDL ratio is the best indicator of heart attack risk and is one of the blood test one should pay attention to. The best ration is 1:1 which suggests that one is healthy.

Weight loss

Adhering to a ketogenic diet plan might be extremely effective for normalizing your weight. However, if one has high fasting insulin, he/she may be required to add a high intensity program (an exercise one). Training has a high effect on increasing the sensitivity of the body to insulin.

What to watch out for on the diet

Disadvantages of ketogenic diet plan are mostly due to its side effects. Some of the side effects are extreme.

Frequent urination

This is because the body is burning the extra glycogen stored in the liver and muscles. This process releases a lot of water which is given out as urine.

Exhaustion and Dizzincss

As the body gets rid of excess water, the body will lose minerals like salt, magnesium and potassium. Lower levels of these minerals will lead to a person becoming tired or very dizzy. This is amongst the well-known side effect of any low carbohydrate diet and the best way to overcome this is to keep replacing the minerals. This can be done by eating leafy vegetables (potassium), magnesium citrate (magnesium) or any other foods that contain the minerals.

Constipation

This is also common with most low carb diets and is usually caused by salt loss, dehydration and magnesium deficiency. This can be controlled by drinking more water and replacing the above minerals

Muscle cramps

This is due to loss of minerals particularly magnesium. It is therefore recommended that a person takes 3 slow discharge magnesium tablets like Slow-Mag for 20 days, and then keep on taking one tablet after wards

Diarrhea

There is need to limit the amount of fat you consume while on the ketogenic diet plan as this results to consuming more proteins. High proteins, low fat and low carbohydrate levels causes signs of "rabbit starvation". It is therefore advisable to replace the carbohydrates with fats, for example, butter or coconut oil and not proteins.

The Building Blocks of the Ketogenic Diet

A ketogenic diet is composed of a variety of foods that have their own health benefits and purposes. Many individuals with specific medical conditions or health goals prefer this diet because of its nutrition as well as having a variety of common foods that don't have to be eliminated from their original diet.

Proteins

A major part of the ketogenic diet is meat because it's the major source of protein. Beef, chicken and fish are important part of the diet because they supply the needed nutrients for the body. For individuals who aren't big fans of meat, tofu is also a great source of protein (and very common among vegans because it doesn't have any animal products). Cheese is also often eaten for its protein benefits but it also has some health set-backs like the high amount of calories and fat, so it's limited in the diet. Many other dairy products that are high in fat are eaten. Whole eggs are some of the most well-known contributors of protein in just about any diet. If possibly, try to purchase range-free eggs and you can also add them to other dishes.

Carbohydrates

Fruits and vegetables are the healthy and most common source of carbohydrates in this diet. Salads with leafy greens, green beans and carrots are the preferable vegetables. Peaches, berries and applause are the most common fruit that can be eaten alone by itself or added to other foods as a topping. Both vegetables and fruits also have many necessary vitamins and can be prepared many different ways, or even eaten uncooked. There are also many pasta substitutes that replace original whole grains, contributing with their nutrients. Spices like sea salt and black pepper also provide this important nutrient.

Fats

Fats compose the majority of the daily caloric intake in the ketogenic diet. They are very important to the body but some fats are very unhealthy and even dangerous to consume, so be cautious. To balance out the nutrients, foods like tuna and shellfish are commonly eaten. Some individuals also like to consume different types of oils (coconut, vegetable, olive, etc.) and add butters to their meat and other foods. Some of the healthiest sources of healthy fat are avocados, but you are also free to try almonds and other delicious nuts.

Beverages

In this diet, dehydration is fairly common so it's important to keep the body functioning properly with liquids. Of course the most basic liquid consumed by practically everyone is water, drink plenty of it! Sometimes coffee will provide a good energy boost as well. All types of teas are welcome, fruit, herbal or others. The more liquids in the body, the better. Liquid sweeteners like Stevia and Erythritol can be added to the tea or coffee for a sweet boost and extra flavor.

The Ketogenic diet is very unique and practically the opposite of the vegan diet. Make sure you consume all the nutrients you need for the day and this diet can have many positive effects on your health and body.

What to Avoid on the Ketogenic Diet

Many methods of losing some weight and maintaining a healthy and fitting body are evolving over time. Selecting the right diet, taking weight loss pills, doing exercises, and surgical methods are a few examples to get rid of excess fat cells from the body. While some of these methods may work perfectly, others may not only have insignificant effects, but also come with side-effects. One of the most effective methods is to practice the Ketogenic diet plan. It is a low-carbohydrate, adequate protein, and high-fat diet geared at burning excess fats. With this low carbohydrate diet plan, the aim is not to restrict intake of calories, but to reduce the amount of sugar and carbohydrate consumption.

What foods to avoid

On this plan, one should avoid food high in sugars, carbohydrates, and unhealthy fats. These diets are not only toxic to the human body, but they also supply the body with excess glucose that is then stored as fat cells. Since they raise blood sugars and insulin levels in the body, it becomes hard for the human body to lose more fats. In addition, human body digests and absorbs food high in carbohydrates faster than in fats or proteins. These processes not only lower metabolism, but also make the person hungry faster than normal, hence increasing the chances of the person consuming more calories that may lead to weight gain. The following is what to avoid on the ketogenic diet at all cost.

Junk or fast foods

These foods do not only contain high amounts of saturated salts and cholesterol, but they also lack essential nutrients the body require to remain healthy. Hot dogs, French fries, and soft sodas are a few examples of these foods. In addition, they contain chemicals and other substances that lower the body metabolism. With low metabolism, the body is unable to burn the food that a person takes, but instead stores it as fats. This effect does not only lead to weight gain, but to other complications such as hardening and narrowing of arteries hence resulting in high blood pressure or diabetes.

Some fruits and vegetables

One should avoid fruits that contain high amounts of carbohydrates. A few examples of such fruits are olive, watermelon, apricots, cranberry, bananas, and strawberry. It is also advisable to avoid the juices that come from these fruits since they do not only contain high carbohydrates, but they also have other artificial addictions harmful to the body. In addition, one should avoid vegetables that grow beneath the earth like onions, carrots, and potatoes for their high carbohydrate contents.

Alcohol

Even though the alcohol may contain no carbohydrates, research show that it slows down the fat burning processes in the body. It is better for one to take free sugar drinks like scotch and vodka, instead of alcohol.

Grain products

It is best for the person on the ketogenic diet to avoid grains and their products that contain high carbohydrates. Examples include white bread, white pasta, what rice, cakes, and pastries. In addition, avoid packaged or processed foods since they contain preservatives and other additions harmful to the body.

Frequently Asked Questions about the Ketogenic Diet

The ketogenic diet was founded in 1920 by Lyle McDonald. It is a very popular diet and is followed worldwide. The ketogenic diet is effective in preventing crises of many kinds as lesser carbohydrates from starches composed of glucose are consumed by the body. After this diet, it is necessary to avoid foods containing carbohydrates like bread, sugar, cereals, pasta and potatoes.

The ketogenic diet has been the staple food for people living in the countryside and also with the Eskimos and many tribes and who basically eat pure protein. During ketosis brain cells are able to get energy from fat instead of glucose. In fact the brain cannot consume fatty acids but uses only ketones or ketone bodies generated during fat metabolism.

Not only is the nervous system not damaged but it has been demonstrated by studies that brain ketosis acts as protective measure against toxic substances like free radicals and prevents hypoxia. Ketogenic diets are recommended by doctors to treat childhood epilepsy or diseases like Alzheimer.

The Ketogenic Diet

The ketogenic diet has been proven to work effectively for a third of patients who become tried and listless after very little effort. Controlled trials have established that a ketogenic diet is found to be effective in the treatment of severe epilepsy in children and adults. Although this diet is very popular among bodybuilders, it does not recommend consumption of foods which are rich in vitamins and minerals, such as broccoli, carrots, sweet potatoes, apples, grapes, raisins, figs, etc.

A Sample Meal Plan for the Ketogenic Diet

Breakfast - Two eggs, two slices of bacon and a boiled tomato.

Lunch - Hamburger meat wrapped in lettuce.

Dinner - Green beans, fried mushrooms and linseed oil with a salmon fillet red peppers.

Snacks - Unlimited yogurt and whole milk, cheese, strawberries with cream, peanut butter.

Frequently asked questions about the effects of a ketogenic diet:

Does the ketogenic diet have negative consequences in the liver or kidneys?

The ketogenic diet or diets based on eating fewer carbohydrates do not have any liver or renal type problems because it is a physiological process for which we are adapted by our own evolution and in fact people who have this type of problems are advised to take a ketogenic diet in many cases.

Is the ketogenic diet carcinogenic?

It has also been shown that the ketogenic diet helps shrink tumours and reduce the percentage of body fat and weight in the most obese people, yes factor that facilitates the development of cancer.

Does a ketogenic diet produce oxidation of cells?

Ketogenic diets increase the antioxidant capacity of the body is increased because oxygenate ketones mitochondria through activation of glutathione peroxidase producing an increase in the synthesis of mitochondrial glutathione. Antioxidants prevent the formation of free radicals thereby preventing oxidation and preventing cell death.

Is a ketogenic diet detrimental to participation in sports?

Many athletes use the ketogenic diet in combination with physical training and use key ketogenic supplements with their diet plan. This obviously needs some knowledge and experience and it is recommended to take the advice from a specialist in ketogenic diets and exercise.

The Ketogenic Diet and Diabetes

Before the invention of insulin in 1920s, the treatment of diabetes relied on dietary control. Diabetics were recommended to modify their diet to control the level of glucose in the blood circulation.

A ketogenic diet is comprised of low-carbohydrate amount. The diet has high fat content that supplements the carbohydrates. Fat is broken down and replaces glucose as a source of energy. The ketogenic diet has only enough protein for body growth.

Less carbohydrate in the diet lead the body to take measures and source for alternative source of energy. The liver releases stored glycogen that is converted to glucose. When the stores are exhausted the body turns to fatty acids replacing glucose.

Proteins are converted to glucose and the body is able to maintain normal blood sugar levels without ingesting carbohydrates. The body can effectively rely on fats for energy functions. Ingestion of insulin is accompanied by health problems. High insulin levels result to weight gain and fat storage sometimes accompanied by heart problems.

A ketogenic diet for diabetics is meant to reduce medical treatment of diabetes. Low carbohydrate in the diet prevents short term effects of diabetes and delays long term complications. The treatment of diabetes requires that medical attention is given continuously. Patients who manage their diet have a better chance of avoiding complications. Low carbohydrate diet leads to the benefit of weight loss and reduces the risk for cholesterol.

When carbohydrates are ingested, the body breaks them into glucose and other simple sugars. The glucose is taken into the blood system. A diet with more carbohydrates leads to toxic levels of blood sugar and the body responds by releasing insulin with the aim of converting glucose to glycogen for storage.

Diabetes occurs when the body does not produce enough insulin to cope with blood sugar after meals. The disease has become common of lately and the solution is to cut on carbohydrates and there will be no need for insulin.

Ketogenic diet is a complement of treatment for diabetes. This requirement of insulin can go as low as 50% easing the treatment procedure. The liver is able to produce glucose from proteins and the brain can rely on this. Some part of the brain only burns glucose for energy. Other parts of the body can rely entirely of fats for energy. With normal fat stores a person can go for days without eating.

Ketogenic diet appears to the body as starvation. The response is reduced insulin production. Oxidation of fatty acids increases to produce energy for body functions.

This method of diabetes treatment is advantageous because it deals with the root source. The aim is to reduce carbohydrates consumption, which is safer than injecting insulin to counteract high glucose level. The diet can be used where insulin is applied and faster results will be observed.

Fighting diabetes can be challenging because of the change in diet and lifestyle. The patients are sometimes mislead and filled with wrong information about the effect of ketogenic diet. It is hard to switch diet just because the doctor recommended. Managing the amount of carbohydrates and medication at the same time can maintain blood sugar for diabetics.

Putting It All Together

I hope you have found this guide to a ketogenic diet helpful and informative. With the proper diet and exercise regimen, you can see incredible changes in your body in very little time.

For any diet to work, you need to take action and stay committed. It is easy to have a cheat day here and there, especially when you are missing your favorite foods, but don't give in to the temptation. One cheat day often leads to another, and you find yourself suddenly not making any progress. Stick with it and believe in yourself. You can do it!

Preview of "Essential Oils" by Emily V. Steinhauser

Essential Oils

Essential oils are oils that are extracted from the flowers, leaves, fruits, peel, seeds, woods, bark, roots, and other natural materials. There are thousands of different kinds of essential oils, and each has unique properties and characteristics. They are highly volatile so they are easily absorbed by the skin. So one wants to take care in the use of them.

Many body care products contain essential oils that they use for their therapeutic properties, and not just for their scent. There are many essential oils that are an effective treatment for a number of different skin conditions. They are extremely concentrated and powerful. They can be regenerative both in physical and emotional ways, making you feel healthy and stronger. The benefits cannot be understated, essential oils can have a dramatic impact on how you look and feel.

This book will explore the various ways that one can use essential oils. I will also present the best oils to use in each specific situation, both from research and personal experience. Sections will focus on the using essential oils to treat, heal, and rejuvenate one's skin. We will also explore how to use essential oils to thicken one's hair, promote faster hair re-growth, and how to deal with hair loss.

Essential oils are often used therapeutically, and I will talk about the medicinal uses of essential oils. I will not only focus on physical application of the oils, but also on aromatherapy and the benefits it provides.

One of my favorite uses of essential oils is using them to deal with headaches, including migraines. They also prove efficacious for first aid, particularly in the reduction of swelling and the healing of bruises. I will also present information on how you can use essential oils to sharpen your mental focus, improve your concentration, and enhance your overall memory.

I am excited that you have joined me on this journey through the essential oils. I hope they bring you a long lifetime of improved health and comfort.

I hope you enjoyed the free preview of "Essential Oils" by Emily V. Steinhauser.

Preview of "Kindle Publishing Secrets Revealed" by James Chen

Learn to Make Money with Kindle Books

Passive income. We all want to make it. And publishing books on Amazon Kindle is a great way to do it. Imagine your books earning money 24 hours a day, 365 days a year on autopilot, leaving you the time to do whatever you desire. Sounds like a wonderful life, right?

It can be, and the first step is publishing your book. This book will guide you step by step through the process, from initial research to how to market your book.

Don't think you are a very good writer? I will show you how outsource your ideas to other writers who will write the books for you. All you need to do is publish them. And collect the checks.

I will also divulge a secret niche which sees extraordinary sales and searches on Amazon. There are very few writers taking advantage of this trick, and those who have are seeing their books in the bestseller lists. The best part: this niche only requires the books be between 15 to 30 pages in length. Short books, huge rewards.

Learn to take advantage of Amazon's enormous customer base, publishing books that will be searched for, found, and purchased. Learn to get your books to stand out from the millions of other ones already available in the Kindle store. It is simple: if people cannot find your books, they will not buy them. Learn how to be found.

The #1 Rule of Kindle Marketing

The rule is simple: find a process that makes money. And repeat it. Over and over again. This rule is particularly effective in terms of Kindle publishing. You publish your book, market it, let it make money, and do the entire process again.

Too many writers concentrate on one book. They invest all of their energy in making it perfect, trying to build up and audience, instead of writing additional books. Understand that having one book found within millions of books requires a whole lot of luck. But if you have two books, your odds increase. Think of each book as a lottery ticket, the more you have, the more likely you will have one hit the jackpot. Your goal should not be to have one book in the Kindle store, but hundreds. Don't imagine yourself as a writer, but as a publisher. And act accordingly.

Authors often focus on the visible success stories on Amazon, on the fiction writers who have sold hundreds of thousands of books. This is an incredibly small group, and their success is hard to replicate, because it was brought about by luck. You will most likely never get this lucky, so you need to create your own success. That means publishing a lot of books.

The people making money in the system are those who publish hundreds of books under different pen names. These books are often outsourced to a group of writers, as are the formatting and cover creation. This book encourages you to embrace the second method and act like a publisher, producing and selling as much content as you can.

Remember the more you publish, the larger your slice of the pie will be.

I hope you enjoyed the free preview of "Kindle Publishing Secrets Revealed" by James Chen.

Other Books Available From Gamma Mouse Media

Below you will find other popular Amazon bestsellers from Gamma Mouse Media.

Essential Oils – Emily V. Steinhauser

Forex Indicators – Warren R. Sullivan

Kindle Publishing Secrets Revealed – James Chen

Procrastination – Warren R. Sullivan

Brain Training Boot Camp – Warren R. Sullivan

Knee Pain Treatment – Emily V. Steinhauser

Marriage Problems – Emily V. Steinhauser

Quiet – Amelia Austin

Lust for Me – Amelia Austin

Cellulite Reduction – Emily V. Steinhauser

The Quick Start Guide to Macarons – Lindsay Stotts

Speed Reading Training – Warren R. Sullivan

Memory Enhancement – Warren R. Sullivan

The Quick Start Guide to Perfect Pancakes – Lindsay Stotts

Compulsive Hoarding – Emily V. Steinhauser

Made in the USA
Lexington, KY
27 October 2014